Poems for Sluts
Kaleigh Gold

Poems for Sluts
Ingram Spark Publishing
Copyright © 2023 Kaleigh Gold
Second Edition
ISBN: 978-1-7382017-0-9

Dedicated to all those who ever used
nasty adjectives to describe me

Table of Cumtents

Slut 1

Seductress 55

Sugar 229

Slimed 357

Afterword 438

Lust is the artist for a canvas full of emptiness

***

"Starting to think
You aren't a good poet
You seduce guys
Steal their poem ideas
And then kick 'em to the curb"
- B

S L U T

Sluts

For years

We have passed along

The common myth

That women

Cannot possess the same level

Of prowess as men

Because it suggests inferiority

So instead

We shame women

Who feel empowered

Sexually liberated

And label these women as

Sluts

This derogation

Comes from a place of feeling

Not good enough

Because these men believe

That a woman used them

And then left

So they devise the notion

That she left because

They weren't good enough for her

She was using them

She could do better

She could find better

From this shame

Echoes a double standard

Because we are so frightened

Of feeling not good enough

That we poison the perception of women

So instead

Of being understood as

Sexually liberated

She is seen as

Tainted

Impure

Dirty

She's such a slut

You hear

Either out loud

Or written on their faces

Eyes full of disgust

Instead of celebrating

The independence

Women fought for

We are cultivated

Indoctrinated

To shame them

Fresh Start

Moving cities

To escape her name

Loathing and vile

And littered with shame

Manipulation

You twirl flirtatious words

Into my hair

With your greasy fingers

Each letter coated

In deceptive adoration

You pierce my skin

With your dauntingly sharp eyes

Like so many pieces of metal

I've jabbed through my skin before

Your silver-tongued suggestions

Overshadowed by idealistic promises

But I'm no naive nympho

You want to mold me

Constrict me

Compress me

Into your version of perfection

Sacrificing my integrity

Scorching my identity

To fit the festering wounds

In your rancid skin

Left by previous women

Substitution

Kiss my neck

Pull my hair

Fill me full of reasons

Why they never cared

Hurting

Society

Pushing me

Up against a wall

Hand up my skirt

Shoving its fingers

Inside me

Reaching deeper

Working me

Like a puppet

Constraints

Bind my hands

Constructs

Duct tape my mouth

Conventions

Strap me to a chair

Customs

Tortured into my body

Sexualized from a young age

Vulgarity

Shoved down our throats

Young girls given no choice

But to succumb to the will

Of stereotypical roles

It's no wonder

We sexualize ourselves

As a means to find connection

It's the only way

We were ever taught

"Early for heels, isn't it?"

Cold morning air

Fresh on her cheeks

Heels against stone

Dim dawn-lit street

U-Hall Girl

"You're her, right?"

What?

No

Not me

I couldn't be

Thought there was a she

Much worse than me

Constantly sleeping

Some new every week

Said she was a freak

100 was her peak

Brought back from bar streets

To her university sheets

But wait

Don't you see

Nasty rumors

Rampantly free

Appalling exaggerees

Feeding hyperbole

Stemming from history

Origin her home city

Always down on her knees

Always caught in a three

Always at some party

Stealing virginity

Voices telling on she

Calling her oh-so-smutty

Disgustingly easy

The grimiest chickadee

Worthless wannabee

Social ejectee

The only merit they see

Is her promiscuity

Delayed Gratification

He twists her golden hair

Wrapping it around her neck

Choking her

Bondage he thinks

While she envisions a noose

Like the one she craved

So many years ago

Now replaced

With a perversion for domination

She wants them to hurt her

Punish her

Hold her down

And spit on her

The self-loathing she once felt

Now manifested

In the form of

Sexual beatings

Pet Named

Sweet cheeks

Sugar tits

Honey buns

Sugar lips

Sweetie pie

Angel face

Baby girl

Cupcake

Sweetheart

Doll face

Puddin pie

Baby cakes

Demanding attention

Demeaning pretension

Lacking dimension

Vulgar condescension

They Know

Purpled knees

Clashing her pale peach

She feels their eyes burning

Assumptions coated in grins

Yeah, That's Her

"I can't believe they hired her"

Reputation precedes

Staff start to whisper

Discussing her deeds

Petting Zoo

They just want to fuck me

Masked behind

Sweet words

Fawning phrases

Romantic promises

But in the end

It's purely physical

You want to use me

Degrade me

Make me your pet

Force your male dominance

In me

Shove your patriarchy

Down my throat

Fill me up

With toxic masculinity

Bar Flies

Eyes burning into my curves

Disgusting fool

Sweet wife at home

Kids my age in school

Weekly Allowance

Bribery

Littering my inboxes

Stuffed full of

Wannabe sugar daddies

Begging to dress me up

Lingerie

Matching heels

Sex toys

Minds with ulterior motives

Fashioning me into a Barbie sex doll

Their throbbing perversity

Charging their credit card

Hush-Hush

Faking intimacy

In a dark storage room

An office chair

Smothered with

Second-hand

Sentiments

Saliva-laced skin

Made smooth

For another

Subliminally

Filling orifices

Like voids

Trauma

Fear me

Respect me

Just please don't

Reject me

Conceal-her

A futile attempt

To cover violet skin

Bruised by lips

Alibi so thin

Afraid of their judgement

Terrified of their thoughts

Peer interrogation

Stomach in knots

Sorry

Silly girl

Don't you know?

They're just using you

For your flesh

Disregarding your thoughts

Too busy tearing their eyes

Into each pink curve

Probing for a way

To remove your walls

Your clothes

Your inhibitions

Strip you down

To your integrity

And yank it away

And you'll be the one

To apologize

Their manipulation

Making you think

It was your idea all along

Carnal

Youthful bones

Teeming with timeless ignorance

They were always led to believe

Sexual fulfillment

Was all they had to offer

In a world full of creative vocations

Their primal purpose was all they served

Assumptions

Shows up to a party

They're huddled in groups

Sees her arrival

They're yelling in troops

"She's here she's here"

Her reputation a tomb

"Who's gonna fuck her?"

"Get her in the bathroom"

No Paparazzi

They fetishize me

I watch their pettish eyes screen

Chest down to where my thighs gleam

Skin crawling

I could just scream

"Slut Sanitizer"

Easy afternoon

Opening bar

Fills up her coffee

Rolling cutlery start

Into the kitchen

Just out of sight

Back to the table

Other servers' delight

Sits at her spot

Sips at her bevy

But ew, what's that?

Chemical taste is so heavy

Turns back around

Sanitizer bottles in hand

Re-screwing on spray caps

Laughter like they had planned

Attention Whore

Always wanting to be seen

Skin barely clad

Outfits obscene

Bright pearly whites

Champagne thread head

Poor doe-eyed girl

Wandering between beds

Fake Rings

False gemstones

Lining both ring fingers

A futile resort

Deterring a disappointing few

Society banded

With moral negligence

Precious metals

Fused with adultery

A seductive inability

To fulfill vows

Wandering eyes

Locked and loaded

With temptation

Eye Candy

Hungry eyes

Grazing bare thighs

Lustful glares

Pulling her hair

Server Grab

They can never keep

Their hands to themselves

Always touching and grabbing

And feeling their swell

Termites

I know what they want

Nasty intentions

Concealed with vague compliments

Disgusting minds

Interrogating my body

Their eyes

Burrowing into my skin

Germy

"Just looking for

A throat to fuck"

Casual

But firm

Just like himself

Objectification

Burnt into his eyes

Derogation

Sewn into his pelt

Daddy's Girl

Cognition spewing from their manhood

Ignorant objectification

Overflowing from their eyes

Probing my skin for naiveté

For a crack within armor

Forged by sexualization

A sickening attempt to pierce me

With their vile fantasies

An ironically sharp contrast

Daughters the same age as I

Inherent paternal protection

From interrogative men

Eerily similar to yourself

Business Meeting

So?

Should I move the car seat from my backseat?

Hair thinning

Liver wilting

Nailing new notches

Into his worn-out belt

On honey

That wouldn't be professional

Promising a ladder to success

Cocaine still fresh

On his dash

WHORE

Written in relish

On her parents' front step

Acid burnt off the sealant

Rain still revealing her rep

NKD Stock

Commodity

Emphasizes worth

Are you valuable

For your assets?

For who you are?

Perhaps we are only

The sum of what we are worth

To others

Do they need you?

Or is exploitation

The only option they have?

                                        "Ugh, fine"

Mind was set

Willpower drained

Tenor syllables

Moaning her name

Legal Age

Impure and insecure

Using sexuality as a mask

Fears and despairs

Validated by anonymous bodies

Numbers to prove self-worth

Self-loathing coupled with peer pressure

An irresistible pairing

For encapsulating emptiness

Sniff Sniff

"What's that I smell?"

Peer voices yell

"A slutty cake-face!"

In junior high hell

Word on the Street

Her name pronounced

With infamy

Hear her coming

Before she leaves

Cover Your Tracks

Always waxed

Mentally cracked

Highly taxed

Publicly axed

Booty Business

Her hair grabbed

With persuasion

Not wanting to

She gave in

Please baby girl

He insisted

Her hands full of

His charcoal sheets

Ouch no I can't

Holy fuck no

Altruistically

Stretching her skin

You like that?

Her answer false

Taught to serve them

Doesn't know how else

Rated R for Reject

You don't become

This slutty for free

Dark nasty things

Tangled history

Rumor Has It

All in the eyes

Sun on her thighs

They all knew she was

Slutty

Critique in their stares

Judgmental hares

Reputation getting more

Muddy

Infamous Name

Sexualized fame

Clinically insane

Devilish acclaim

Historical shame

But it's the name of the game

When your libido's to blame

"Then get out"

Dark street

Dead phone

Kicked out

All alone

"But it's his birthday"

I don't care

Don't want to fuck you

Too impaired

Wandering down

Lamp-lit streets

No home to go to

When you're this "slutty"

Neuralyzer

Wanna come in?

And fiddle my fin?

My sweet violin?

Make me fizzle

Deep within?

Baby boy

Just spit on my sin

Push your tongue

Deep within

Make me forget

Just for a min

All the horrid things

That I was pushed in

Golden Roast

Here's a toast

To our favourite roast

The girl with the most

Holes as the host

Slut-Shamed

Shouted halls

Playground brawls

Bus home hauls

Classroom walls

Email trolls

Handwritten scrawls

During kickball

Late night calls

Tripped footfalls

Excluded dance halls

Hiding in stalls

Called her too small

Lanky and tall

Nose a bird call

Blubbering know-all

Slutty neanderthal

Freaky odd ball

Insults that appall

Slipping downfall

Going awol

Mental cell walls

Kicked out in rainfall

Abusing alcohol

Constant pub crawls

Resort to eight-balls

Drug free-for-all

Black-out waterfall

Numbing protocol

Suppressing recalls

Emotional stone wall

Stuck in pitfalls

Disgusting catcalls

Sexual tetherball

Exploited rag doll

Craving to end all

Down the wormhole

No farther to fall

Final roll call

Heel Clicks

The lonely socialite

Traipsing up and down the avenue

Searching for reality

Searching for a clue

Past Life

She lets the first glass

Slide down easy

Too easy?

Almost as easy as herself

Or at least

How she used to be

High School Blues

3 am

6 missed calls

7 boys she knows from school

2 of them sucked

2 of them fucked

And all won't leave her alone

Over and over

Her phone goes off

She's sick of picking up

Leaving her voicemails

Filled with such hatred

Telling her to finally off

Kill yourself

You worthless slut

It echoes through her mind

Malicious laughter

Fills her rafters

Maybe she'll take their advice

SEDUCTRESS

Fatal Femme

Carcinogenic woman

Scratching her claws into your skin

Soaking your bones in seduction

Filling each pore with toxicity

She'll consume you

From the inside out

Lapping up your serotonin

Gnawing on your complacency

Slurping up your tired veins

Pushing remnants of trauma

To the side of your plate

Stomach full of soul

She'll abandon your desecrated corpse

Lucid rotting flesh

Scented with succubus pheromones

The deadliest disease

To leave you alive

Digits

How silly of you

To assume

You were anything

But a number

Another notch

On my invisible bedpost

Sleeping

Where so many others have

Once you step out that door

Your memory becomes

Purely numerical

Cinematography

She's always pursued

A preoccupation with sexuality

Her mind

Bound in ropes of lust

Her libido

Thrusting against her

Since youth

While other's minds are bemused

With keen ideas

Hers

A pornographic reel

Dirty desires

Course content

Film saturated in skin

Locked n Loaded

Manipulative mind

Tongue fill of venom

Stars in her eyes

Her lips as the weapon

Reckless Lust

Ignorant to your ramifications

They tell you

You hurt them

You don't care

Already infatuated with your next kill

But you lie awake

Alone

Stewing in the consequences

Of your deep-seated

Commitment issues

Not afraid to be loved

But terrified

Of loving someone else

Honey Cinnamon

Expensive haircut

Silver temples

Gaudy ring

Pushes a button

Darling come in here

Adjusts his tie

Winks

Boys;

Carmela

She's leaning in the doorway

Caramel

Skin

Hair

Eyes

Cream silk draped

Against her satin

Lashes framing fox eyes

Sun-kissed freckles

Laced on sin-kissed skin

"You called?"

Velvety smooth syllables

Slipping off red lips

Gold chain

Dripping down her chest

Seduction

Pooling in her collarbones

Ravenous eyes

Nipping at each curve

Carnivorous thoughts

Probing her skin

Hands balled in soft fists

Contracting muscles

Wanting to taste her name

Craving to taste her batter

Spirited Away

Merlot machete

Bordeaux blade

Baby boy come over

Let's misbehave

Take Heed

Lock his eyes

Weak his knees

Invade his mind

Seduce with ease

Say you'll give him

What he needs

Make him beg

Make him plead

Suck his lips

Please baby please

Rotten darling

You're such a tease

Rip his hair

Feel him breathe

Crush his soul

Death by triple D

Corrosive

She's toxic

A noxious nectar

Volatile by all means

Regality seeping from every pore

Next

Eye them

Smirk them

Cheek them

Flirt them

Warn them

Lust them

Break them

Crush them

Can't Say No

Seduction in her eyes

Perversion in her grin

Nasty thoughts in thigh-high socks

Sipping on her gin

Medusa

Name derivative of cunning grace

Paralysis cursed into her eyes

Ravishing beauty turned serpentine

Peer into her blues and fossilize

Dungeon Dragon

Eyes full of sin

She fills them with gin

Bites at their skin

Corrodes from within

Her mind full of malice

They'll drink from her chalice

Alone in her palace

Seeking self-solace

Brick House

Energy dripping

From her fingertips

Intelligence shining

From her sassy quips

She'll wink her blues

Then eat the vic

Stone cold prize

But her heart's

A brick

Falling Short

Maybe she doesn't

Let them in

Because none of them

Deserve it

No Plus One

Are none of them

Good enough?

Or perhaps your boxes

Are in excess

Your generation

Now marrying

And you're still

A desolate mess

Careless Bear

But she never called them

Because she didn't care

Soon to be forgotten

Once hacked from her lair

I Spy

From across the room

I grab their gaze

With my own

Eye fucking them

As hard as I can

I hope they can tell

I like it rough

I stare into their soul

Their masculinity gets hard

To ignore

With my ocean blues

I'll reach into their psyche

Pull out who they are

Embody everything

They desire

It's all a façade

Silly men

Don't you know

I'm just using you?

Manipulative bitch

With a libido

That just doesn't quit

Camouflage

Dirty blonde

Teal blue eyes

Cocky smirk

Dreamy guise

Hardened Criminal

A sickening passion

For smashing

Breaking hearts

Turned to ashen

Used to be

Broken

Bashed in

Now combing streets

Lacking compassion

Barricade

Eager fingertips

Reaching across her skin

Little do they know

She'll never let them in

Heard You the First Time

Quit saying "omg"

I get it bud

I'm a different broad

Insatiable thirst

And likes it raw

Eats your heart

And makes you watch

Practice

Eye fucking herself

In the mirror

Sex in her eyes

Gaze in her guise

Intentions getting much clearer

Reverse Squirt

"I've only seen that in porn"

I know my dear boy

I felt it in your legs

Novelty quivering through your core

Garbage

Forgive me father

For I have sinned

I've sat and watched

Their filthy grins

Perversion in my

Every whim

They're lost

I've found them

'N filled them with gin

Licked toxicity

Deep in their skin

Pushed them back

Then pulled them in

Pumped their guts

Blood mixed with sin

Hurt them good

Then ditched 'em

In the bin

                                                    Pass it on

Emotionally withheld

Historically unwell

Commonly misspelled

Sexually compelled

Rubber Ducky

She's slick

She's clean

She's squeaky

She's mean

Killer Queen

Plunging neckline

Bare nails

Plunging the knife in

Pink entrails

Taste his past

Sweet berry wine

Won't let them pass

Before they whine

Tripped

Baby boi

Just take a dip

Reach inside

Get a grip

GF Material

She's slimy

& grimy

& loaded with sin

She's toxic

& noxious

& corrupt from within

Harsh

She never had her heart

On her sleeve

Stone cold chest

Unwilling to reprieve

Her own worst critic

Mirror kissed with shame

Notorious syllables

Comprising her name

Virulent Vixen

Succubus skin

Spitfire sin

Grind on their grin

Corrode from within

The Villain

Have men always been this awful?

Rhetorical interrogation

Paired with a $9 sav blanc

Swirling with frozen raspberries

Drowning her doubts

In introspection

But darling

Is there a common denominator?

Champagne blondie always on the run

From any healthy rapport

Perhaps men are not as awful

As you have been to them

Silent manipulation

Seething from her glassy eyes

Corrosive exploitation

Dripping from her tongue

Indulging herself with the audacity

Of blaming her shortcomings on men

Read at 10:38

A toxic tendency

To give up with ease

Ignore their pleas

Silence that frees

Pizza Box Sharpie Note

Wake up

Strange couch

Strange ceiling

Strange sounds

Lips dry

Mind fogged

Memory

Liquor logged

Should I leave?

Should I go?

Leave him here

On his own?

Would it be rude?

Would it be nice?

Waking up alone

Are you surprised?

Plead Your Case

"Sit on my face"

But does he deserve it?

Get on your knees

Beg baby worship

Fire Tongue

Baby girl

Do you learn?

Spitting harsh words

Filled with cold burn

Willfully ignorant

As they yearn

Callous nonchalance

Making them churn

And She Never Saw Them Again

Oh she

Knew how to date

Caught in her eyes

Losing their gait

Waltzing away

What a good night

Daydreaming 'bout

Her sweet little tight __

Sex Trophy

Selling her paintings

To past lovers

Trading nostalgia

For yet another

Harder - on Herself

Perfectionist eyes

Carving her skin

Narcissistic gaze

Probing within

Hopeful

Hopes thick with gin

Hope lining their grin

Hopes on nervous skin

Hope dripping down their chin

Cum Laude

Left university

With a degree

In infamy

Trained skillfully

A mastery

Of unsympathetic

Promiscuity

Devil Woman

She's done a lot of shit

With a lot of guys

Stole their hearts

Fucked their eyes

Starry eyed

She sucked their souls

Dragging their emotions

Through red hot coals

Last Supper

Listen here boy

Eyes full of tease

Do what I say

Get on your knees

Slick perverse hands

Grabbing your hair

Making you beg

Making you swear

Back to the floor

Thighs to your ears

Baby you want it?

C'mon let's hear

My lips on yours

Grinding your grin

Skin dripping wet

Skin full of sin

Watermelon

Juicy skin

Filthy mind

Eat his flesh

Leave the rind

Flip it 'n Reverse it

He says he'd let me

Peg him

On international women's day

And who said

Chivalry is dead?

Hardened men

Silently begging

To be dominated

In bed

Mind Control

Drool on their lips

As she starts to strip

Obsessed with her hips

Can't help but drip

Listen Up Punk

Honey baby

Can't keep his dick

Out of my hands

Oh you want more?

Obey my commands

Easy A

Down the hatch

And up her snatch

These boys all think

They're quite the catch

But what they don't see

And what they don't know

Is how easy they are

You've just got to blow

Coaxed

Her lips coated in gloss

Dress far too short for a boss

But she's in his head

Wants her in his bed

Craving to coat her in sauce

Jaw Grab

Who's your mama?

Eyes cocked

Thighs locked

His eyes full of fear

Head shocked

Heart rocked

Made all his fears

Disappear

Carnivore

Filthy flesh

Between her teeth

Feels so good

Makes him weak

Nameless

Messages littered

Unsaved contacts

Don't care to know you

Spitting harsh facts

Forgotten

Getting over them?

Not even a second

Lock eyes

With the next

Then she'd go

And she'd wreck 'em

Dismissed

Contention

Dressed in seduction

Mal intentioned

Obsession with rejection

Bite Me

Intimacy

You dance with it

Like a rattlesnake

You want it to bite you

Let it suck blood

Out of your flesh

But you're afraid

Terrified

Of the pain

Of it pulling away

Leaving you alone

A wreck

You'd rather feel agony

Than nothing at all

Phantom Ganon

His lips smeared

With her ruby gloss

Finally got the courage

To battle the boss

Female Gremlin

Pussy rockin

Coochie throbbin

Tongue be mobbin

Throat game goblin

Carefree

Freckled skin

Sun-kissed palms

Eating their hearts

Without any qualms

You Are

Cause she looks like sugar

And she talks like rain

Whisper in his ear

And he's already came

Smell her on your skin

And you lick up her name

Can't get enough

And who's to blame

Poppet

Control freak

Make him squeak

Make him claw

Make him speak

Push Back

You don't want me?

Not if I don't want you first

Rejection caught in her grip

Chasing an unquenchable thirst

"We just don't vibe"

A common message thread

But it really isn't them

She just lives in her head

Petrified of transparency

Brick walls to appear tough

Terrified that they'll discover

She doesn't believe she's enough

Tailored

Weeding out the ineffective

An arduous task

Tossing them aside like rubbish

Along with her custom-made mask

Battle Royale

Sapphire eyes

Spit fire sin

Claws in her gaze

Fighting their whims

Dommy Mommy

Well well well

Look who it is

You again

Couldn't get enough of me?

You perv

I bet you thought of me all day

Didn't you?

Holed up in your tiny office

Jacking off under your pathetic desk

Imagining being suffocated

By my massive tits

Gasping for air

Getting drool all over them

You disgusting little man

You like that?

I'll give you something to think about

Go home and touch your wife to it

Sicko.

Emotional Moat

Don't let him in

Don't let him win

Runner's High

Run for cover baby

Cause I'm gonna get cha

Bite my teeth right in

And really fuck wit cha

Grab you in my slick grip

And start to mess wit cha

Suck your soul clean out

Then run away from ya

Let's Play Cranium

Prides herself

On giving the best head

It's all that she's heard

Moaned from her bed

Chick Flick

Narcissistic

She's sadistic

Hyper quick chick

She's a sick bitch

"See ya round cowboy"

Her messages littered with

Cookie cutter rejections

Beyond practice

Now habitual

She isn't sorry

Justification seeping from

Her wandering eyes

Abandonment

Dressed in flirtatious nonchalance

Not afraid to break them

But petrified

Of vulnerability

Cracked Artifact

Mentally detached

Romantically unlatched

Historically unmatched

Sexually abstract

On Your Knees

God you're hot

What's your damage?

He can keep up

But she's totally savage

A picture of him

And she's practically famished

Beg baby plead

Do you think you could manage?

Donkey + Dragon

Fire in his mind

Ice in her heart

Begging for reprieve

Doomed from the start

Throat Glock

Whitened teeth

Eyes that read

Seduce with ease

Disrupt the peace

Make him plead

On her knees

Can barely breathe

Elbow grease

Ineffective

Hard woman

Soft dick

Either that

Or he cums too quick

"Yes, I promise"

They don't believe

Her either

Crumpled up napkin

Unseen digits

Thrown in the trash

Shortly after

Enticing Icing

Style before comfort

Hips encased in leather

Barren legs reflect sunlight

Regardless of the weather

Borderline Abuse

Coupla of dimes

Fake furs the bar

Eying up men

That don't meet their bar

Tossing sarcastic smiles

But the guys won't get far

They only want men

Who take it too far

Red Flag

Confusive

Elusive

Abusive

Delusive

Meaty

Although

I've never been much

Of a meat eater

I've always been

A carnivore

Hunting down

My next kill

Ravenous in anticipation

Longing for a taste

You fill my mouth

Gagging on flesh

Choking on skin

Feeding an insatiable appetite

Picture Perfect

Esmerelda

She's a curse

She'll make you sick

Then hurt you worse

Turquoise hair

Dark teal eyes

Gouging her nails

Into your thighs

Strike Attack

The spark of novelty

Gleaming in her iris

Timed execution

By her prefrontal gyrus

Gold Widow

She only replies when she feels like it

Eleven men wrapped around her pinky

Dozens more caught in her web

Hundreds trapped in her gaze

She doesn't care if she hurts them

Only infatuated with the concept

Of being the one that got away

Goosebumps

Golden hair

Sultry stare

Long legs bare

She doesn't care

Catalyst

I want to hurt you

Beat you

Bruise you

Turn up the heat

Unglue you

Make you yell

Make you moan

Scar you with reasons

Make you grow

"Are there others?"

I'm hot and single

Honey of course there are

You wanna join 'em

And be my cigar?

Anti-prude

She's lewd

Crude

Usually partially nude

Her mood?

Sultry attitude

Sometimes a bit rude

Manipulates dudes

Often deludes

Using her nudes

To sexually exude

Her love to get screwed

Orange Juice

A catalyst for destruction

Leaving them in the dust

A wrecking ball

Thrashing against glass

But instead of windows

Emotions of others

Her ignorance

A lead pipe

Smashing hearts

But in the destructive ruins

She stands alone

Surrounded by wreckage

A graveyard

Of love interests

Beaten to a pulp

Flashback

Sickening daydreams

Carved into her skull

Her dangerous libido

Holding the awl

Scratch it in darling

Before you forget

Etched into her thoughts

Bodies writhing in sweat

Irish Exit

I make them seem

Like it's too good to be true

And then I leave them

Before they realize

It isn't

Wild Cat

Eyes red

With lust

Hunger

Searching for the next victim

Devour him

As if you're starving

Begging for your next meal

His skin

Ripe with innocence

Thick with naiveté

Much easier to impress

To use

To abuse

Caught between

Infatuation with power

And an addiction

To the terrified look

In their eyes

Soul Sucker

She scribbles her name

With her tongue in cursive

Right on the tip

Coercively perversive

Sexual Exploitation

Flirtatious initiation

Seductive intimidation

Motivated inebriation

Graphic imagination

Willing participation

Phallic manipulation

Deliberate concentration

Sublime copulation

Physical annihilation

Mortal disambiguation

One-sided interpretation

Idealistic romanticization

Habitual negation

Purposeful delegation

Selfish justification

Emotional frustration

Begging desperation

Mental incarceration

Vengeful emasculation

Bucket List

Wrapping her legs

Around his desires

Daydream

Deja vu

Sick Son of a Bitch

You want me to sit on your face?

My juicy ass cheeks

Suffocating your every breath

How about I grind on your lips

Pushing my skin against your teeth

I'll make you lick me

Top to bottom

Forcing your tongue inside me

As I water board you

With wetness

Ask and you shall receive

Puma

Her name in his mouth

His stuff in hers

Blonde in his hands

Making him purr

Playbook

Rumination

Dripping out of every orifice

False pretension

Seeping from her lips

Cerulean eyes

Covering lies

Darling when will it end?

Emotional Dildo

And before

They could anticipate it

I'll leave

I'll say it's me

It's not

It's always them

Unfulfilling

Unsatisfactory

Just a piece of meat

That couldn't fill the void

Oops

Open purse

Grocery store

What's inside?

Vibrator

Expendable

Why chase him

When you could

Replace him?

Scrolling

Messages

Littered with unnamed contacts

I don't care to know

Who you are

A distant memory

(If you're lucky)

Of a drunken night

You think you're special

Don't you?

"I'm not like other guys"

Or so your mother

Led you to believe

But the hundreds of messages

Lining my inboxes

All eerily similar

Would beg to differ

Sorry for using you

For a drink

A shot

Entertainment

An escape

Perhaps we had chemistry

But we'll never know now

Lost in an iMessage sea

Of good intentions

And willful ignorance

Unperturbed

All of these lovers

Toxic

All of this nonchalance

Noxious

H2Hoe

Cold water glass

Placed on the nightstand

Warm him up good

Then give him the grand

Gulp down some icy

Trapped in your mouth

Drag your body down his

Tease your way south

Pout the bottom lip out

Slide it up his him

Water starts to dribble out

Lock his eyes

Lock his skin

Slowly mouth over the tip

Roll around don't even think

Throat it all then look at him

Swallow

Wink

                                                    Meow Mix

Kitty too good

Kitty just right

Kitty on his mind

Playing in the moonlight

Toxic Traits

She likes to leave

Before she is left

Arm's length

So they can't climb her walls

They can't hurt her

Since she won't let them in

Emotionally withheld

So she'll never fall

Cradle Robber

Your baby blues

Echo naiveté

I grab your heart

With my icy fist

You succumb to my will

Performing anything

To please me

Cockpit

Red lipstick

Not a dipstick

Sassy quick wit

With some sick tits

Sex Water Bottles

Want some water?

Words trying to catch their breath

Their skin streaked with sweat

Icy cold glass

Crowding the fridge door

Wine bottles in a previous life

Parched fingers fiddle

For the lid

Just as countless others have

Can't Stay

Faint handprints on her door

Reminiscent of him

Begging for more

Venomous Woman

Infecting men with her gaze

Sickening seduction

Poison flowing from her fingertips

The taste of her lips?

Tantalizing

The feel of her skin?

Paralyzing

Her leaving without a trace?

Unsurprising

  Using

Musing

Abusing

Amusing

Perusing

Sleepover?

A familiar flair

To rearrange her bedroom

A perverse preference

Grown from waking up to strange ceilings

Winter Woman

Heart of ice

Lips of snow

Frost-bitten men

Get used to the cold

Succubus

Thighs pressed with lace imprints

Their naive tongues

Fresh on her freckled skin

Shitty kissers

Still burnt into her tongue

Her tight hamstrings

Nailing their hearts into her bedpost

Brass printed with provocation

Sheets stained with oxytocin

It's Not Me...

No no

Dear sweet mess

If I'm too much?

Go find less

One-track

Erotically charged

Sexually driven

Preoccupied mind

Hair in a ribbon

Sick vulgar thoughts

Surging her brain

Eyes rolling in

Carnally insane

Ditched

Thoughts trippy

Attitude lippy

Mind full of crime

Sexually sublime

Devour your guts

Leave you in the dust

Music

Filling her up

Pounding each cavity

Vibrations resonating

Echoing through each chamber

Every cell

Bathed in bass

Benadryl

A taste of your own medicine

You hate it

Bitter like hotel coffee

Scouring your taste buds

Like his tongue did

Who knew medicine

Could make you feel

So sick?

4 Hours Later...

Smile at the people

Down on the street

Coffee in hand

Sun on their cheeks

Only hours ago

Filling his needs

Making him hurt

Making him scream

Melting Point

She loved the power

The fire within

To exert control

Temptatious sin

Unleash the wrath

Then cut him thin

Boil his neurons

From the outside in

La Petite Mort

Quick wits

Huge tits

Obsessed with

Making them sigh

Pink lips

Subtle nips

En Français

She'll make you die

Poetically Uninspiring

Sorry honey

You just didn't do

Couldn't inspire me

Couldn't cut through

Brick walled heart

Silver slick tongue

The nastiest thoughts

But emotionally numb

Drop Off

Sorry darling

There isn't a spark

Go play with the boys

Out at the park

It's not me it's you

So sorry for this

I don't wish you well

No thanks to the kiss

Social Buffet

Grip in her grin

Spit on her chin

Toxin within

Eats on a whim

Wicked Witch

Lips like honey

Skin like sin

Eating out their hearts

Chipping their chin

Guile Smile

She's vile

Hostile

Agile

In style

Profile?

Versatile

A beguile

Crocodile

"You fuck like a thirty-year-old"

His leg tremors audible

Between each syllable

My neighbors likely wondering

What "holy shit" x 20

Was regarding

Or perhaps they know

Fairly little is surprising

In this day and age

Stone Wall

Devoid of emotion

Intangible commotion

Eyes like the ocean

Saliva like potion

How the Turn Tables

Well well well

Look who it is

The man who can't

Keep himself

Out of my biz

Looking well

How have you been?

Aversion in her eyes

Seduction in her grin

C.E.HOE.

Make them work for it

Make them beg

Show them who's boss

Legs like nutmeg

Mmm Salty

Soft

Sensual

Seductive

Strong

Eats your

Heart

Then licks

Your palms

Double-edged Whore

Hurt me first?

Do your worst

Couldn't even

Make me squirt

Hurt you back

I'll be your curse

I'll make you ache

Until you burst

6 am

Dim lobby lighting

Ass on the floor

Lacing her heels

Snuck out the door

Knight Moves

Using her body

As a physical barrier

The usual defense

None shall pass

Emotional barricade

Sexual fortress

They Think They Know Her

Giggly golden-graced girl

Viciously vivacious vixen

Egocentrically enticing enchantress

Selfishly salivating siren

Rattle

Her blood was like venom

Poison in her veins

Infectious

Corrosive

Burning anyone

Who dared to get close enough

Teaser Pleaser

She does this thing

Where she doesn't put out

Heightens their hopes

Tightens the rope

All Together? No.

Vodka soda

Silver black hair

Light in his eyes

Holes in his ears

Should we go blaze?

Hope in his smile

Food in his teeth

Blood in his thighs

Sorry I can't

Gotta go home

Pack up my lunch

(Leave me alone)

A change in his tune

Hurt in his eyes

Just separate bills

"I guess we don't vibe"

Sprint Mobile

Come on baby

Don't be a chore

Ignite my mind

Don't be a bore

Talking to you

Should always be fun

Unless it isn't

Then darling I'll run

Rocky Start

Stone woman

Granite gaze

Igneous eyes

Metamorphic maze

Diamond heart

Limestone lips

Regards you as

A pebble chip

Fall/Winter

She'll choke you

Till you're barely breathing

Think she wants you?

Changes her mind like a season

Femme Dégoûtant

Preoccupied mind

Swimming with impurities

Her fingers eager

Her vision hazed

5 inches of stiletto

Deep in his jugular

Blood on black leather

Red bottoms soaked in crimson

Light draining from his eyes

Soul leaking from his veins

And ugh

Doesn't it feel good

To get back at (his name)

Boo

Ghosts from my past

Knocking at my door

Buried skeletons

Asking for more

Beta 'Blayground

Craving an alpha

To tear off her dress

To smash up her guts

Leave her room a mess

Bitter Medicine

Six foot ~ish

Gelled over hair

Joggers and Nikes

The fuck boy stare

"I'm not like them"

His personal brand

Manipulation by iPhone

Trying to steal your hand

You know all his tricks

He leaves you on read

Succumbed to his will

Thinking about him in bed

Little does he know

He's in the same trap

Fuck girl extraordinaire

Curled up in his grasp

Mask Up

Icy eyes

Peachy thighs

Silken hair

Sultry stare

No Choice

Smash mat

Crash pit

Flirt so hard

They had to hit

Notebook

Can I write in it?

Innocence on his lips

Ignorant to my aversion

Babbling on about irrelevancies

I don't care to know you

Locking eyes

With men at other tables

You don't know me

And luckily

You never will

Take a Picture

Chai on her tongue

Champagne in her hair

Golden skin barely clad

Addicted to their stares

Dark Horse

She's better in

The dark

Light eyes

Cold heart

She's meaner than

His last

Dirty mind

Thoughts crass

High Bar

Afraid of her strength

Destined to be alone

Can't fuck her right

Can't get in her zone

Mommy Dearest

From boys into men

She showed 'em the ropes

Took 'em round the bend

And gave 'em the stroke

White Toes?

Might be a hoe

Loves to fuck

On the hardwood floor

Asking for it

And they give her more

Tastes so good

Tastes like a whore

Pineapple juice

Like it's her chore

Tosses men aside

If she gets bored

Brainwashing

Her name's Desire

Reaching in through their eyes

Eye fucking their souls

Licking their minds

Sucking their coals

Cronch

Blondie destined

To be someone

From above her eyes

To below her thighs

Just a character

From the start

Soon to be tearing

Unsuspecting hearts apart

How'd she do it?

She'd wink and kick ass

Stabbing men in the heart

Crunching bones with sweet class

"Is anyone sitting here?"

An endless parade

Clowns without paint

Politeness doesn't work

I was never a saint

Swing Batta Batta

Bleach blonde

Beach bomb

Batting hearts

With napalm

Level: Rock Hard

She's that next level up

Type of girl

The one who steals your heart

Hurt so good

It'll make you hurl

Vibrato

Eye contact is crucial

When you're doing dirty things

Grab onto his pupils

Then suck till he sings

Hungry?

Petulant kisses

Dance at his hips

Surly torment

Waltzing across his lap

Her velvet shimmied down

Lapping at her bones

Taunting his appetite

Dangling meat above the bone

Horsey

Follow his rhythm

Adapt to his needs

Ain't got no rhyme?

Overpower that steed

Sought After

Baby girl

Don't forget who you are

You make them swear

And they come from afar

Impossible to ignore

They just can't resist

Always caught in your hair

Begging for your wrist

Caulk Talk

Leg lock

Hip rock

Shake to make

His squawk gawk

Zomb

Sexually charged

Erotically driven

Eating cold hearts

Not considered living

Amusing

But my dear sweet boy

You must have known?

You're just a muse

You're just a clone

Of all the men

Who've pushed and pried

Spitting soft words

How hard they've tried

And now you lay

In messied sheets

Creative inspiration

Only temporarily

Been There, __ __

Flashing eyes

Darting gaze

Wanted you once

But never again

Svetlana

Privet babies

I am here to teach you lesson

You want man to love you? Yes?

No.

You want man to n e e d you

Without you?

He dies.

So darling,

You must appeal to his physical senses

His needs

His primal desires

Sight?

You dress up for others

You already impressed him darling

Dress for those who would be interested

If he was gone.

Sneaky yeah?

Taste.

Everyone knows

Man's heart is in stomach.

So feed him

Learn his meals

Make them better,

Don't show him how

Smell.

You like when he smells good?

Him too.

Let him know before you enter room

With his nose

Perfume dictates mood

Got it?

Sound.

He needs your voice in his thoughts

But not regular voice,

Sexy voice

Softer, slower, deeper

You know what I'm talking about

And lastly; touch.

Man needs to feel you on him

Give him something to fantasize about

Grab him

Hold him against your breast

Feel his breath

Pull him in,

Graze your lips across his

Look him in the eyes

And whisper,

"Dinner's ready"

SUGAR

Good Gravy

Your pretty words

Press into my skin

Carving each syllable

Into my bones

You trace your fingers

Down my spine

Your silky touch

Sears into me

How could simple pillow talk

Resonate so deeply

Within my physical body

Quick n Dirty

Closed off

Show off

Lights on

Clothes off

KFC n Booze

Ocean eyes

Battered thighs

Buttery lips

Take a nip

Like a gin

Soaked in sin

Lick me up

Flesh corrupt

RIP

Moonlight-soaked sheets

Two racing heart beats

Lust covered breath

Fuck me to death

Oxytocin Mask

Hungry eyes

Sin-kissed thighs

Matted hair

Gasping for air

Dewy

Glistening skin

Pinky flesh

Soaked sheets

Your sweat

Traced under

My fingerprints

Your pores

Open from

The heat

Foggy window

Panes coated

In condensation

Gravity

The words roll off my tongue

Right onto your lips

Cascading down your chin

Licking at your hips

Twilight Tango

Navy blue sky

Night beyond young

Satin peachy thighs

Dance on his tongue

Gustatory Gratification

Roll me in your palms

Like clay

Mold me

Knead me

With your fingers

Squeeze my flesh

Between your teeth

Taste me

Like blood

In your mouth

Bite me

As hard as you can

Am I salty?

Or sweet?

Sugary skin

Etched

Into your taste buds

Imprinted

Onto your tongue

Engrained

Into your mouth

Branded

Into your hippocampus

Oh you'll remember

How I taste

Saturated

Feel me cum

On your fingers

Digits sopping

With chemical intensity

Sidetracked

Hands on her

Legs on him

Fingers curled

Around her gin

Pretending to listen

Mind occupied

Thinking about

Him sliding inside

Candyland

Lips like sugar

Eyes like coffee

Tongue stretched words

Legs like toffee

"You're a biter hey"

His salty skin

Between my teeth

Incisor marks

Deep in his sheath

3rd Degree

Your lips ignite my skin

Burning imprints on my flesh

Fiery kisses

Imbedded into my thighs

Your tongue scorching hot

Pillow Talk

Sugary words

Coated in lust

Infatuation

Drips out of our pores

Your grey sheets

Already soaked

You tell me I'm perfect

I say I'm just me

And that's enough

He kisses into my mouth

You don't love me

You just love what my body does

False feelings

Saturated in passion

Infused into one night

                                                    Come 'Ere

Fingers trembling

Sparkling thighs

Muscle contraction

Back rolling eyes

Wasn't Listening

Words laced with suggestion

Glazed eyes tracing each other

Teeth gnawing on their lips

Minds sidetracked with sexuality

Throat Hockey

They're hiding

In the hall

Outside the

Bathroom stalls

Grins above

Their jaws

Seduction in

Their cause

Charlotte?

Thighs intertwined

The dance has begun

Licking intents on their lips

An enticing web they have spun

Blessings

Bow your head

Say your grace

Eat this kitty

Off your plate

Vertebraid

Closed lids

Bodies entwined

Serotonin swimming

Up our spines

Musical Genius

Your pulse beats against my neck

Innate percussion

Reverberated by my own

Each thrust harmonized with mine

A melody of our muscles contracting

A symphony of skin contact

Rhythmic breaths echo euphony

Each of us a conductor

Of this orgasmic opera

Nailed

Smacked up

Scratched up

Yank my hair

Gashed up

Pushed down

Pulled in

Spread my legs

Full in

Christopher Throbbin

Winnie baby

Come lick my honey pot

Fingers in deep

Uh yeah that's the spot

Zapped

Eyes wide

Thighs pried

Arms tied

Mind fried

Get a Whiff

Your scent

Soaking my sheets

My olfactory lobe

Doused in your

Pheromones

Sucker

Suck on me

As though

I'm flavored grape Lick

me like a lollipop Suck

the sugar out Saturated

saliva

I always knew

You had a sweet tooth

Mechanics

Look inside

Feel my drive

Look alive

Lick my vibe

Careful

Suck my skin

Pull my hair

Make me shake

Make me care

Serpents

Speakeasy

Orange leather

His tongue on mine

The taste of cocktails

Slithering through our entrails

Feisty fingers

Slinking up my skirt

Likewise

Easy eyes

Butter thighs

Sultry guise

Midnight skies

Step Up

Please handsome

Won't you fuck me on the stairs?

Rug burn on my knees

Hurried hands in my hair

Solo Performer

She's gnawing on her lips

Like she wants him to

Visions of their thrashing bodies

Dance between her thoughts

Memories coated in sweat and fluids

Slipping down her hand

Sexualized daydreams

Pushing her to the edge

Aftermath

Swollen lips

Reddened thighs

Messy hair

Starry eyed

Ignition

Torch my skin

Ignite my mind

Light my lips

Burn my spine

Comfy Couch

Green velvet

Thighs on thighs

Sneaky digits

Wet surprise

Winded

Hands in her hair

Stealing all her air

Devilled Legs

His silver tongue

Smears persuasion

Across her skin

Drag it once

And she'll cave in

Bubbling Up

Tub overflowing

Suds on the floor

My legs on his

Lock on the door

Flesh Right

Cashmere skin

Velvety smooth

Buttery and pliable

But strong and supple

Your silky satin slips

Beneath my fingertips

Creamy peach

So juicy

I can't help but taste it

Jelly Jam

I shake my thighs

For the look in your eyes

I bounce my cheeks

Just to make you feel weak

Doors Locked

The dashboard lit

By dim streetlamps

The dull glare of the moon

On the windshield

Kissing you in the darkness

Feels criminally good

Indulging only my senses

Of taste and touch

Iris Virus

Reach into my eyes

Pierce my pupils

Grab my gaze

With yours

Eat me up

In the blink of an eye

Chipotle Mayo

Nasty intentions

Fingers covered in sauce

Dragged down your tongue

Now you're the boss

"Can you get the zipper?"

Numb lips

Bruised hips

Cheek dips

Unzipped

Good Hussle

Power hour

Golden flower

Flesh devoured

Hit the showers

Lip Smacking

Gustatory bombardment

On my mind

Sexual involvement

Consuming my time

Canny

Between your thighs

I taste into your eyes

Reaching into your mind

Devouring skin

Like an addiction

Gardening

Feel the ground beneath your palms

Dirt the colour

Of coffee with cream

Use your nails to carve your name in

The softest earth

Dig in with your fingertips

The soil already soaked

Dig deeper

Then

Press your hard shovel

Into the earth

Penetrating as deep

As the flower bed

Can handle

Cradling

Hardened Norse hands

Wrapping her thighs

Slick tongue singing

Sweet lullabies

Unlaced

Encompassing sexual tension

Unlike ever before

Brawny fingers inside her

Lingerie thrown on the floor

Numbing Agent

You press your lips against mine

Seduction nestled into every crease

Saliva infused suction

Weakened at the knees

Funetics

Your name

In my mouth

It rolls off my tongue

Each syllable

Savored

3rd Degree

You skin scorches mine

Igniting it

Wild like fire

Hot to the touch

I can't get enough

Searing my senses

My tongue

Immediately charred

Urgency

Gnawing on skin

Muscle between teeth

C'mon baby boy

I need you in deep

Car Lickness

Staring at the streets

Her taste in his teeth

His tongue on her cheek

He's taking the lead

Anticipation

Pores exuding sexual charisma

Fingerprints carved in with lust

Eyes brimming wide with intention

Thighs dripping with musk

Filthy Animals

Writhing bodies

Sweating against each other

Copulation dripping

From each orifice

Pores soaked

In adoration

Pink Slip

Something new

On her lip

Supple skin

Against her hip

Water's fine

Take a dip

Lap him up

Take a sip

Midnight

Dashboard lit

City glare

Caught his hands

In her hair

Milkshake

He's disrespecting

Her makeup

She's causing him

To shake up

I Scream 4 Ice Cream

As a child

My favourite flavour

Was tiger tiger

But I suppose now

Yours must be papaya

Licking up my ice cream

Savoring every second

Sopping up the heavy cream

With your rose-tinted taste buds

Papaya

All over your lips

Lick until you can't anymore

Thrashing

Wrapping his hands

Around her throat

Making her squirm

Making her choke

Greenroom

Desecrated couch

Legs long past gone

Fluids falling beneath hot thighs

Only used as a sexual pawn

Lock Jaw

Grab my hair

Shake my head

Ruin my muscles

Tomorrow's dread

D8 Night

Secondhand shirts

Smiles then he flirts

Hands up my skirt

Intentions like dirt

Pleaser

Fingertip

Tip toe

Up and down

Your spine

Losing grip

Hip throw

Make you feel

Divine

Internal Percussion

Rhythmic bass

Drumming our tympanic membranes

Our muscles

Contracting to the beat

Symphony infused sweat

A melody sugar sweet

Lightening Kisses

Pried lips

Closed lids

Pressed against

Walls with skids

                                    Safety Meeting

Tip of my tongue

Let's have some fun

Eyes merge to one

Stop drop and run

Pounce

Dim lights

Hazy drinks

Slick tongued

Saucy minx

Mindful

I want to feel your skin

On mine

Your body pressed

Against mine

Your heartbeat paired

With mine

Your pores sweating

On mine

I can't help it

Your mind

Constantly

On mine

Gore Whore

Turning in the mirror

Eyeing all the scratches

Skin beneath your nails

Sexually infused gashes

Theatre Darling

Onyx sheets

Center stage

Dynamic action

Passionate rage

Eyed Up

Grab my skin

Seize my gaze

Lost in our glare

A cerulean maze

Dirty Smirk

Thinking things

She wouldn't dare say aloud

The good

The bad

The devilishly evil

Craving his skin on hers

His sweat in her

Torn

Shoved against the seat

Calluses in her hair

Ripping at her neckline

Giving her the stare

Bruised Peach

Bad habit

Hypnotic eyes

Eat my flesh

Bruise my thighs

Taste Test

Suck on my skin

Pull out the sweat

With your tongue

Fill my pores

With your saliva

Grimy and delicious

Salty and addictive

Sweetheart

Tongue tied

Bodies pressed

Hands held

Kissed with zest

Negronis?

Infecting my skin

With his gaze

Liquor-ish memory

Staring to haze

Echo Chamber

Thighs entwine

Oxytocin sublime

Felt his him

Pulled him in

Reverberations

Deep within

Lost @ Sea

Crashing into each other

Like waves

A roaring sea of lust

Drowning the both of us

Immersed in passion

Soaked in sex

Parked on a Football Field

Curly hair

Filthy stare

Midnight glare

Lip locked lair

Lips so right

Muscles so tight

Feel his fight

Sweat at night

Swiss-Chz

Our bodies

Speaking in tongues

He's licking my lips

Skin sopping with saliva

Dainty nails piercing sheets

Sorry

"I want to write the whole book"

He tongues into my mouth

Taking cautious care

To lick the tips

Of my teeth

Nightcap

2 am

His cologne on my skin

Sweat in my pores

Tongue soaked in gin

Scalding

Grinding my lips

On yours

The taste of my flesh

Burning holes

Through your tongue

"Let's go for a drive"

Wring her neck

Curve her back

Taste her smile

Midnight snack

Temp Agency

Sure

Not a forever

But maybe

Just a for now?

Kisses

Sweet like nectar

Until you have to say

Ciao?

Grime

Scratching impurity

Into my skin

Filling my nasty guts

With disgusting sin

Fruit Basket

Blueberry eyes

Pink peachy thighs

Strawberry lips

Papaya hips

Your Treat

Making him bend

Making him sway

Making him purr

Did it his way

Sheet Havoc

Clothes

Strewn on the floor

Scotch glasses

Fingerprinted and unfinished

Weed

Filmy across the air

My lips

Raw and chapped

It's strange

To find comfort

In such disarray

Don't Stop

Back against metal

Hips against his

Baby hit the pedal

Make my insides fizz

Animalistic

Pouncing tigers

Emerald eyes

Glimmering golden

Soaking thighs

Smooth like jaguars

Rich dark sheets

Tantalizing tangles

Magenta cheeks

Dick in a Box

He's up against her thighs

Rolling back his eyes

Biting teeth like knives

Get ready for the surprise

Reflection

Your name

Melting in my mind

Like coffee creamer swirls

The taste of your skin

Caught behind my eyes

My tongue rolling

In a curl

Spanky Panky

Cinnamon sugar n spice

Bodies are shaking like dice

Baby don't think twice

Didn't come here to play nice

Bees Knees

Roll me around

With your tongue

Making me beg

To get stung

  Picasso

Prussian blue

On her back

Clothes strewn

On the floor

Painted thighs

Greedy eyes

Don't stop

Give me more

Sweetie

Honey kissed

On my lips

Sugary sweet digits

On my hips

Night Drive

Moonlight

Bouncing off the dash

Your lips

Pulsing at my neck

Collarbones

Dripping in desire

Red light

Your curls between my fingers

Tongue

Between my teeth

Heat between my

Thighs

Green light

Cummy Bears

Rippling like butter

Trailing down my chin

Locking our eyes

Making him twinge

Candid Camera

Apartment pool

Water bottled merlot

Back against tile

And he's pushing so slow

Daydreaming

In her mind

On her tongue

Licks her lips

Comes undone

Cheshire

Hands on her

Lips on him

Feel her purr

Deep within

Marked Up

Ripping his skin

Tearing his sheets

Soaking his thighs

Filling his needs

Secret Meeting

Darkened office

Speakers aflare

Whispering nothings

Temptatious air

Shawty Fire Burnin

Heat in his touch

Fire in his grip

Torch in his tongue

Charring her lips

Sailor Jerry

Incisor marks on his ear

Pink nails across his neck

Thighs curled into the couch

She's grinding on his deck

                                                    C*ck R*ck

Lip lock

Tick tock

Head knock

Skin shock

Hot Shoulder

You bite his flesh

Like a meaty rib eye

Gnawing on muscle

His salty skin

Fills your mouth

His deltoid

Stifles the moans

Ugh

Leather against glass

Greedy lip against lip

A fistful of blonde

She's starting to drip

Rare

Steak in her guts

Craving

Steak in her guts

Filet mignon

Choice grade A cut

Fill me up baby

'N make me your slut

Circle of Thrust

Dress at her hips

Tempt on his lips

Lust in her grip

Illicit ellipse

Whatever You Want

Saliva nectar

Running down

Her limbs

Sweet divine

Submission to

Every whim

Fruitcakes

Nuzzling nectarines

Prismatic peaches

Fluorescent figs

Oxytocin screeches

Focus Mode

Lips on him

Mind on him

Thighs on him

Sighs within

Crave TV

Cocked brow

Smirked eyes

Tongue just begging

For a filthy surprise

Re-reading

Sliding into

Her thoughts

Oxytocin assassin

Name swishing

Through her teeth

Habitual habanero

Charring her tongue

Sugary sweet

Recollections

Glued to her screen

Mental projection

The highlight reel

On replay

An infatuation

With his

Cinematography

They say

The eyes are

The windows

To the soul

But perhaps

They give insight

Into the toll

That each word takes

A crippling addiction

To raspy vocal breaks

It Slipped?

Honey baby

That wasn't the plan

Thighs in my grip

Blonde in his hands

Lights Off

Inside your

Mind

Tasting your

Rind

Blackness without

Blind

Unhinged by

Time

Immersed in the

Sublime

Dirt Squirrel

Leaning in to kiss her

She spits in his mouth

Feels the heat beneath her

Scratching his way south

Touch Me

Freshly shaved legs

Yearning to be grabbed

Glistening with coconut

Craving masculine nails

To pierce into supple softness

Calloused fingers imploring

Her vanilla-traced hamstrings

SLIMED

11 am Walk of Fame

Sleep deprived eyes

Ringed with smudged liner

Whites reddened from

The front row splash zone

Cheeks still traced with him

Wave to the nice people

On the street

S is for sex

Sucking on skin

She's soaked in saliva

Smearing his spit

Suggestively

Sensually stimulating

Sugary sweet satisfaction

Seductive sentiments

Swimming between

Slimy

Slithering skeletons

Spicy as salsa

Soft as satin

Sexuality

Scorching their skulls

Artistic

Corrupt my flesh

Saturate me in sin

Sexuality dripping

Down my legs

Let me taste myself

Your tongue

Painting with spit

My skin

The canvas

1000 Ways to Die

I grab the bed sheet

Nearly ripping it in the process

My fingers and toes curling in

Deeper and deeper

I can barely handle it

My bite marks

Visible on your pillow

You hold me down

By my neck

Forcing me to take it

Harder

It's like you read my mind

I can barely breathe

Gasping between moans

Asphyxiation never seemed so hot

Harder

Plus forté

Mas fuerte

Durior

Piu forte

Schwerer

Tezê

Kovemmin

Sil 'neye

Trudneijsze

bent v fingers

Ooga Booga

He drags his fingers

Across his wet tongue

Saliva webbed between them

Locking his eyes with mine

He touches me

With such cruel intensity

A monster

No longer beneath my bed

Now biting

Between my legs

Specimens

Hickeys on her tits

Swollen like a fish

Pushed into her splits

Bed a petri dish

Muddy

I'll lick you up

You filthy mess

Suck out all the grime

Dirt between my teeth

Nasty and disgusting

Mud all over my face

Impurity all over my chest

Creamed

Yikes

What was that?

Stand up

Kumquat

Cum shot

From playing all that

Hopscotch

Soaked crotch

From her squishy soft spot

Ventriloquism

Something healthy

Brushing her fingertips

New adoration

Kissing her tits

Her mind strung up

Like a marionette

Another hand inside her

Making her wet

LSDF

Lick me

Suck me

Dick me

Fuck me

Authority

So fucking hot

Perhaps that's why

A man in uniform

Becomes that much more

Irresistible

Pierce me

With your bossy gaze

Lock my eyes

With yours

Feed me

Commands and orders

I'll do anything

To prove my worth

Bending over backwards

For your approval

Drops of Jupiter

In her hair

On her face

Dotted on her chest

Spraying astronomy

All over her bed

Sheets lit like stars

"Did I say you could stop?"

His nails

Digging into my neck

Fingers threatening

Asphyxiation

Each thrust

He bears down more

Cutting off

My air supply

Don't stop

Crush my windpipe

Who needs air

When suffocation

Feels this damn good

Crazy Horse Girl

Never was into horses

But damn boy

I want to ride you

Break you in

Riding your pink lips

Grinding your meaty hips

Untamed stallion

Succumbing to my will

Who's your equestrian?

Tye-Dye

Your tie

Hurriedly wrapped

Around the doorknob

Too bad

I was hoping you'd

Tie me up

I guess instead

We'll just have to

Race across

The finish line

Or will it be

A tie?

Bang Bang

Thick flesh in her nails

Hot spit on his tongue

He's going faster

He's shooting his gun

Smut Slut

You want more?

Filthy whore

Begging to get fucked

On her bedroom floor

Not enough?

Oh you'll get it rough

Hands like weapons

Skin so tough

Robo Sex

I've been a bad bad cyborg

In need of some servicing

Come over and tune me up?

Grab me by the fuse box

Rewire my circuits

With your metal digits

Feel my metal

With your automated tongue

Rearrange my machinery

With your hard drive

Spray hot oil

On my nasty joints

Overheat me

Crash my operating system

Maybe then I'll learn

To be an obedient AI

Victimized

Dick in her mouth

Wink in her eye

Convulsing on her bed

He's ready to die

Deadly

The tip of the tongue

The teeth

The lips

Spit on her skin

Drool on her tits

A sucker for punishment

She won't make it quick

Thirst in her eyes

As she eats his __

Destructo

Touch my sweat

Taste my heartbeat

Bite my skin

Tear my bedsheet

Finger Sandwiches

Go on

Take a bite

Just a nibble

A morsel

If you will

Use your hands

Devour me

Put me on a table

Eat me

Off the fine china

Smash me

Like a plate

Take out your anger

Your trauma

Your bruised history

On the dishes

Throw me to the ground

Make the hurt go away

Scattered

Like broken shards

On the floor

Nice Carrot

Asthmatic

Jack rabbit

Fuck me once

Make it a habit

Fresh Meat

Best drunk sex

You've ever had?

Filled with tequila

Bodies unclad

Baby boy

Put it in

Fill my guts

Make me sin

Soaking sheets

Nasty smiles

Out of breath

Seductively defiled

Asphyx

Gagging on you

Just another way

You choke me

Barely breathing

Saliva forced

Down my throat

Begging for

Annihilation

Blacklight Nightmare

Her floor

Littered with clothing

Furniture soaked in sweat

Their writhing bodies

Leading a path of destruction

Handprints streaked on tables

Leather slick and clawed

Ignorance fueled by lust

Lollipopped

Soaked in saliva

Spit trailing from her lip

Eyes rolling back

His reality ripped

Brutality

Break my neck

Yank my hair

Fracture my spine

Cut off my air

Skull Fucked

Hands nasty

Fingers grimy

Lips vicious

Tongue slimy

Hair pulled

Jaw locked

Spit soaked

Throat cocked

Eggy Leggys

Brain fried

Sunny side

Tongue tied

Dirty ride

Corked

Daydreaming of ways

He'll make me shut up

Fill up my mouth

And force me to suck

After 8

Power top?

Or power bottom

Lock my legs

'N I've nearly got him

What's my name?

I want to hear

Lick your lips

Moan in my ear

Breathe in my sweat

Sexually asphyxiate

Cum for me handsome

Cum sometime after 8

Baby Come Back

Sexual innuendos

Painted all over the walls

Stains between sheets

Provoking withdrawal

Adjectives

Filthy

Nasty

Sweaty

Sticky

Dirty

Grimy

Nitty

Gritty

Cum Here

He whispers

His curled fingers

Pressing her

From inside out

In and out

Like fucked up clockwork

Pulsating

Pushing her to the edge

Metacarpals and Phalanges

Wrap your hands

Around my throat

Choke me

Dig your nails

Into my porcelain skin

Spread your fingers

Though my aurelian curls

Grab me by my hair

Yank it

Spread your fingers wide

Pull back

Slap my ass

As hard as you can

I want to feel

Your skin connect with mine

Stinging flesh

Use your hands

As punishment

Make me hurt

Make me pay

Make me learn my lesson

Make it Count

Carpe my diem

As hard as you can

Grab a hold of me boy

Then seize till you can't

Hysteria

Come here baby

Don't be lazy

Just obey me

Don't say maybe

Get on the bed

Let's get wavey

Rip my skin

And turn me crazy

Punching Bags

Nails piercing his shoulders

Scratches carved into his back

Pummeling her senseless

Her organs under attack

Sex Liquids

Lube

Streaked in her hair

Spit

Running down her chin

Sweat

Dripping down her face

Cum

Filling her throat

Conductor

Fingered grip

Calloused hands

Make her beg

Filled demands

Pushed her closer

Soaked her skin

Played her like

A violin

Mother Pucker

Suck me like a sucker

Fuck me like a fucker

Super Soaker

Surfs up dude

Riding you

Like the waves

Using my limbs

To hold you down

Under the tidal wave

You've caused

Dousing you

Drenching you

Drowning you

Feel the liquid

Squelching between

Our grinding bodies

                                        Jackson Pollock

Sexual dexterity

Explicit mortal gain

Perverse artistry in her eyes

Raspy tenor painting her name

Tick Tock

Baby girl

Just wants to dance

Let loose

And drop her pants

Find a man

To bend her stance

Fuck her right

And fuck her fast

Willpower

Hands wrapping my throat

Spit smeared on his skin

Thighs contracting now

He's slowly giving in

Neck Snap Crackle Pop

Your sweaty fingers

Curl around my blonde locks

Yank

My head ripped back

As I'm thrust forward

Ouch

I should have known

You don't care

About my spinal health

Dibs

Squeeze my flesh

Bite my lip

Push in hard

Ownership

Me Me Me

Wine me

Dine me

Pick me up

And 69 me

Hold me

Fold me

Slap my ass

And scold me

Eat me

Meat me

Use your hands

To beat me

Flirt me

Hurt me

Now you're gonna

Squirt me

Conference Call

Aged walnut

Coated in gloss

Black nameplate

And you're the boss

Expensive pens

Pushed aside

My back on the desk

And you inside

Verbal Filth

High socks

Thick cock

Bruised knees

Dirty talk

Choose Your Weapon

What's your favourite colour sweet cheeks?

Rubber?

Silicone?

Let's get you a toy

He mouths into mine

His tongue articulating

Inside me

Reaches under his bed

Sliding drawers

Impressive

8 inches of black

Meaty fingers

Yanking my peachy thighs

To the edge

Eye fucking me

Like a premonition

Licks the longest three fingers

Warms me up

Then

Ugh

Alright do your worst

Salty Sweet

Him

All in my mouth

Swish don't spit

Saltwater rinse

Apple Bobbing

He grabs a hold

Of her hair

Meaty fingers

Pulling and pushing

Her blonde strands

Like a leash

Gasping for air

Liquid

All over her face

Down her throat

Desperate for the prize

Egged On

Animalistic

So sadistic

Voyeuristic

Antagonistic

Nympho

Vehicles

Trampoline

Bathrooms at parties

Grocery store parking lot

Car hood

Elementary school tarmac

Elevator

Classrooms

Fenced dumpsters

University dining hall

Furnace room on patio cushions

Elementary school field

Playground trees

Bar bathrooms

Ravine party woods

Yoga studio

Friend's mini van

Side of a friend's house

Music festival stage

Club alley

Common room couches

Communal showers

Hooker hotel

Storage office

Apartment building pool

Kitchen floor

Recording studio

Cafeteria hall

Thirsty

Push down with your tongue

Slide side to side

Push against my bone

Wet

Is an understatement

Sop it up

With each drag of your tongue

Suck on me

As if you're parched

And I'm an oasis

In the Sahara

Demander Gentiment

Je veux m'etouffer sur ta bite

Jolie s'il-vous-plaît?

Safe Word Off

No rules in here

Every night is purge night

Slaughter me sexually

Black sheets

Soaked in immorality

                                    Counter-cock-wise

Peel them off

Lightly grazing

Him

With your fingertips

Lick your hand

Then slide it down

Spit on the other hand

Double duty

Hands twisting

Spit trickling down

Your tongue

Pressing up from the bottom

Drag it to the top

Swirl

Then take it all

Aren't you a hungry girl

Roughin It

Heavy calloused hands

Grab your legs

Flip you over

Grabs his t-shirt

Ties you up

Your hands

Trapped behind your back

He hooks a leg

Into each elbow

Yanks you

Your face

Buried in sheets

His meaty fingers

Grab your ass

Like two handles

And then

Ugh

Fuck

Corn Shrub

Won't you come over

And watch porn with me?

My mirror

A plasma flatscreen

Parallel to the bed

We'll make our own

Amateur hour

Canvas Stretching

Dig your claws

Into my flesh

Hurt so good

Make it stretch

Short Circuit

Scratch my itch

Feel me twitch

Hit the switch

N make me glitch

100% Tip

Locked metal door

She knows the code

Scrambling inside

Sexual mode

Backs up against

Dry storage shelves

Teeth biting lips

Their baddest of selves

Hand up her apron

Fingers inside

Nails in his neck

She's liquified

Spins her around

Ass in both hands

Tray as a weapon

Blonde beside cans

Marionette

Go on

Slide your fingers in

First one

Then two

As far as they'll go

Move your fingers

To make the puppet talk

Up and down

Round and round

Your meticulous fingers

Make the puppet dance

Faster

Put on a show

Don't stop

The puppet

Writhing

Manipulation

Into the finale

Gym'n It

Hot

Breathing

Sweaty

Lifting

Intense

Slipping

Steamy

Gripping

Humid

Heaving

Dirty

Dipping

Wet

Staining

Cardio

Training

Main Floor

A dangerous game

We play in here

The elevator rising

Sex driven by fear

My hands pressed against

Silver stainless steel

Fuck me faster

Before somebody hears

Christmas List

What do you want, little girl?

If you're good

He'll hand deliver it

Get on your knees

And pray for it

He'll creep in at night

And give it to you

Like you want it

Like you've begged for it

Hoe hoe hoe

Get your jollies

Script

Ugh yeah

Like that

Don't you dare

Stop

Yeah?

Ugh fuck

Yeah

Oh my fuck

Don't stop

Yeah

Yeah?

Yeah

Ugh

Yeah

I'm gonna

Mmm

Yeah

Oh my god

Yeah

Holy fuck

Hardware

Shoved against her workbench

Hard wood

Pushing against peach (skin)

Heavy hammering

Reverberating her bones

The harder the better

Flipping over

Nailing some more

Finish the job

Screwing tighter and tighter

Her skin covered

In elbow grease

Blasted

One

Then two

Three

Not four

Curl your fingers

Make me beg

For more

Breakfast?

Ugh

Peachy skin pushed into marble

Feeling him in between me

Grabs my waist

Then my

Ugh

I'm under his fingers

Put down the spatula

Grabbing his neck

With my nails

Slides me sideways

Stone flush with my stomach

My saliva coated palm

Grabbing him

Begging for it

His fingers dig into my shoulder

And then

Ugh

Water Board

Temptation traced lips

She's asking for it

Seduction-soaked eyes

Thoughts gushing with grit

Back against satin

His tongue on her skin

Suffocation by choice

Saliva trail to his chin

La Fin

So now you know

The life that I've lived

The things that I've did

The ones I have tripped

Grown from pride

To ignorance

But now

I simply admit

What's done

Is done

Now move on

Let live

Afterword

The contents of this book span the last ten years of my life. In high school, the material began to write itself.

Since my early teens, I have turned to writing as an outlet to process my experiences. The good, the bad, and the horrendously ugly. Thousands of memories have been strewn out in ink and typed out on screens.

Many of these poems were difficult to put into words. The first chapter - SLUT - was particularly tough. Rehashing trauma and manipulating it into beautiful language takes a toll; regardless of how much processing has been done. The final poem "High School Blues" has been written over and over - and deleted over and over. I never wanted it to be part of my collection, even though it was a pivotal point in my life. Rather than succumbing to the encompassing pressure to end my life, I kept moving forward.

I knew the strong seductress I was meant to become.

As for all those who unknowingly collaborated with me, I appreciate your minds, bodies, and words. Guinea pigs and instructors alike, you have been instrumental in my process.

I am grateful to be able to share these experiences with you. Whether you relate to them or not, I hope they have granted you insight into the secret lives that women live and the foundational experiences that shape emotional and sexual development.

About the Author

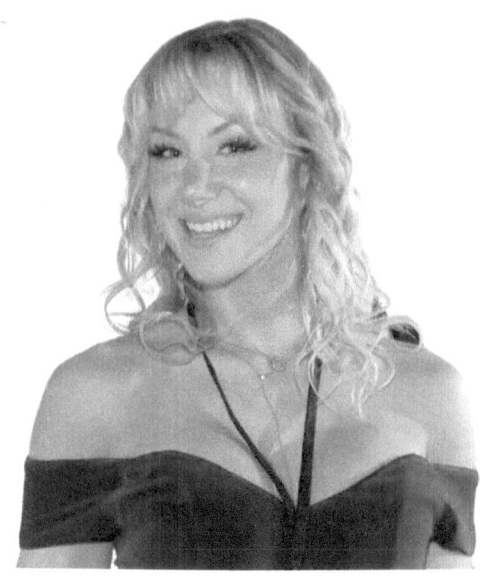

Kaleigh Gold is a Calgary-born artist who dabbles in writing, painting, and Speech-Language Pathology.

When not entwined in poetically transcribing her thoughts; she is likely to be covered in paint, reading a Stephen King "phatty", or cooking up something fierce in the kitchen.

Her love for language emerged early in adolescence, extending into a near expulsion in university for writing essays paid for by other students. She then went on to study Speech Language Pathology with an emphasis in Autism Spectrum Disorder and Childhood Apraxia of Speech.

Catch her next book, *The Mentally Illest*, Fall 2024.

Thank you for your time, your thoughts, your compassion.

Now let's move forward and make sexual liberation the norm.

Always with love,

KG

www.ingramcontent.com/pod-product-compliance
Lightning Source LLC
Chambersburg PA
CBHW022042160426
43209CB00002B/43